MW01224182

WHO Global Report on Falls Prevention in Older Age

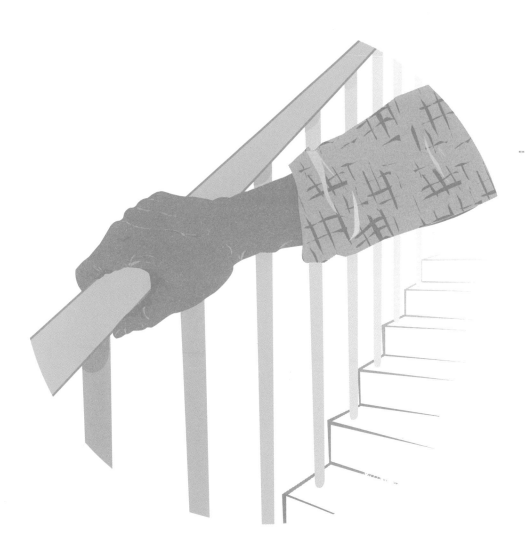

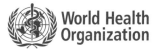

World Health Organization

WHO Library Cataloguing-in-Publication Data

WHO global report on falls prevention in older age.

1.Accidental falls - prevention and control. 2.Risk factors. 3. Population dynamics. 4.Aged.
I.World Health Organization.

ISBN 978 92 4 156353 6   (NLM classification: WA 288)

Design: Langfeldesigns.com Marilyn Langfeld/Art Director, Adina Murch/Design,
© Ann Feild/Didyk Illustration

Contents

Acknowledgements

This global report is the product of the conclusions reached and recommendations made at the WHO Technical Meeting on Falls Prevention in Older Age which took place in Victoria, Canada in February 2007. The report includes international and regional perspectives on falls prevention issues and strategies and is based on a series of background papers that were prepared by worldwide recognized experts. The papers are available at: http://www.who.int/ageing/projects/falls_prevention_older_age/en/index.html

The report was developed by the Department of Ageing and Life Course (ALC) under the direction of Dr Alexandre Kalache and the coordination of Dr Dongbo Fu who was closely assisted by Ms Sachiyo Yoshida. ALC would like to thank three institutions for their financial and technical support: the Division of Aging and Seniors, Public Health Agency of Canada; the Department of Healthy Children, Women and Seniors, British Columbia Ministry of Health and the British Columbia Injury Prevention and Research Unit.

The contribution and input of the following experts are gratefully acknowledged: Dr W. Al-Faisal (Syria), Ms Lynn Beattie (U.S.A), Dr Hua Fu (China), Dr K. James (Jamaica), Dr S. Kalula (South Africa), Dr B. Krishnaswamy (India), Dr Nabil Kronfol (Lebanon), Dr P. Marin (Chile), Dr Ian Pike (Canada), Dr Debra J. Rose (U.S.A.), Dr Vicky Scott (Canada), Dr Judy Stevens (U.S.A), Prof. Chris Todd (the United Kingdom), Dr G. Usha (India) and Dr Wojtek J. Chodzko-Zajko (U.S.A.).

Editing, layout and printing of the report was managed by Mrs Carla Salas-Rojas (ALC).

Chapter I. Magnitude of falls – A worldwide overview

1. Falls

Falls are prominent among the external causes of unintentional injury. They are coded as E880-E888 in International Classification of Disease-9 (ICD-9), and as W00-W19 in ICD-10, which include a wide range of falls including those on the same level, upper level, and other unspecified falls. Falls are commonly defined as "inadvertently coming to rest on the ground, floor or other lower level, excluding intentional change in position to rest in furniture, wall or other objects".

a) Problems in defining falls.

The adoption of a definition is an important requirement when studying falls as many studies fail to specify an operational definition, leaving room for interpretation to study participants. This results in many different interpretations of falls. For example, older people tend to describe a fall as a loss of balance, whereas health care professionals generally refer to events leading to injuries and ill health (1). Therefore, the operational definition of a fall with explicit inclusion and exclusion criteria, is highly important.

2. Magnitude of falls worldwide

a) Frequency of falls.

Approximately 28-35% of people aged of 65 and over fall each year (2-4) increasing to 32-42% for those over 70 years of age (5-7). The frequency of falls increases with age and frailty level. Older people who are living in nursing homes fall more often than those who are living in community. Approximately 30-50% of people living in long-term care institutions fall each year, and 40% of them experienced recurrent falls (8).

The incidence of falls appears to vary among countries as well. For instance, a study in the South-East Asia Region found that in China, 6-31% (9-13) while another, found that in Japan, 20% (14) of older adults fell each year. A study in the Region of the Americas (Latin/Caribbean region) found the proportion of older adults who fell each year ranging from 21.6% in Barbados to 34% in Chile (15).

b) Fall injury rates.

The rate of hospital admission due to falls for people at the age of 60 and older in Australia, Canada and the United Kingdom of Great Britain and Northern Ireland (UK) range from 1.6 to 3.0 per 10 000 population. Fall injury rates resulting in emergency department visits of the same age group in Western Australia and in the United Kingdom are higher: 5.5-8.9 per 10 000 population total.

c) Need of medical attention.

Falls and consequent injuries are major public health problems that often require medical attention. Falls lead to 20-30% of mild to severe injuries, and are underlying cause of 10-15% of all emergency department visits (18). More than 50% of injury-related hospitalizations among people over 65 years and older (19). The major underlying causes for fall-related hospital admission are hip fracture, traumatic brain injuries and upper limb injuries.

The duration of hospital stay due to falls varies; however it is much longer than other injuries. It ranges from four to 15 days in Switzerland (20), Sweden (21), USA (22), Western Australia (23), Province of British Columbia and Quebec in Canada (24). In the case of hip fractures, hospital stays extend to 20 days (25). With the increasing age and frailty level, older person are likely to remain in hospital after sustaining a fall-related injury for the rest of their life. Subsequently to falls, 20% die within a year of the hip fracture (26).

In addition, falls may also result in a post-fall syndrome that includes dependence, loss of autonomy, confusion, immobilization and depression, which will lead to a further restriction in daily activities.

d) Fall mortality rates.

Falls account for 40% of all injury deaths (27). Rates vary depending on the country and the studied population. Fall fatality rate for people aged 65 and older in United States of America (USA) is 36.8 per 100 000 population (46.2 for men and 31.1 for women) (28) whereas in Canada mortality rate for the same age group is 9.4 per 10 000 population (29). Mortality rate for people age 50 and older in Finland is 55.4 for men and 43.1 for women per 100 000 population (30).

Figure 1 (page 3) shows fatal falls by 5-year age group and sex (31). Fatal falls rates increase exponentially with age for both sexes, highest at the age of 85 years and over. Rates of fatal falls among men exceed that of women for all age groups in spite of the fewer occurrences of falls among them. This is attributed to the fact that men suffer from more co-morbid conditions than women of the same age (28). A similar difference in mortality between men and women has been reported following hip fracture. The incidence of hip fracture is greater among women while hip fracture mortality is higher among men (32). One study found that men reported poorer health and a greater number of underlying conditions than women, which substantially increased the impact of hip fracture and consequently increased the risk of mortality (33). Or is it not that men who fall have more co-morbidity than other men in general.

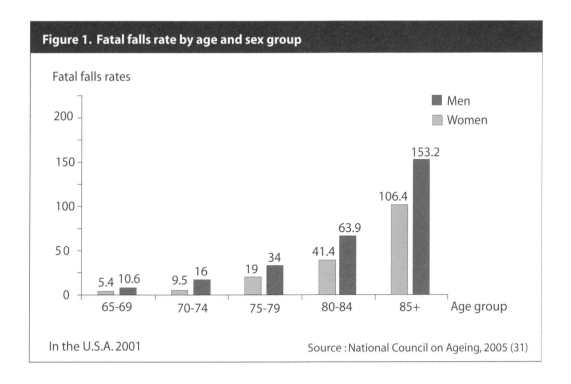

Figure 1. Fatal falls rate by age and sex group

Fatal falls rates

■ Men
■ Women

In the U.S.A. 2001

Source : National Council on Ageing, 2005 (31)

3. Population ageing

"Population ageing is a triumph of humanity but also a challenge to society" (34). Worldwide, the number of persons over 60 years is growing faster than any other age group. The number of this age group was estimated to be 688 million in 2006, projected to grow to almost two billions by 2050. By that time, the population of older people will be much larger than that of children under the age of 14 years for the first time in human history. Moreover, the oldest segment of population, aged 80 and over, particularly prone to falls and its consequences is the fastest growing within older population expected to represent 20% of the older population by 2050 (35).

Figure 2 illustrates the population pyramid in 2005 and 2025. It highlights the growing proportion of older population in parallel with a decreasing proportion of younger population. The triangular population pyramid of 2005 will be replaced with a more cylinder-like structure in 2025.

a) Impact of population ageing on falls.

Falls prevention is a challenge to population ageing. The numbers of falls increase in magnitude as the numbers of older adults increase in many nations throughout the world. Falls exponentially increase with age-related biological change, therefore a pronounced number of persons over the age of 80 years will trigger substantial increase of falls and fall injury at an alarming rate. In fact, incidence of some fall injuries, such as fractures and spinal cord injury, have markedly increased by 131% during the last three decades (36). If preventive measures are not taken in immediate future, the numbers of injuries caused by falls is projected to be 100% higher in the year 2030 (36).

This applies to many developing countries where currently close to 70% of the elderly population lives, and where population ageing is occurring rapidly. "Unlike the developed world that became richer before getting older, developing countries are getting older before becoming richer" (37). This is reflected in the fact that health in older age is neglected in some developing countries. Falls prevention is one of the issues that have not been given a sufficient attention. For instance, there is a lack of epidemiological data in many regions of the developing world.

4. Main risk factors for falls

Falls occur as a result of a complex interaction of risk factors. The main risk factors reflect the multitude of health determinants that directly or indirectly affect well-being. Those are categorized into four dimensions: biological, behavioural, environmental and socioeconomic factors.

Figure 3 encapsulates the risk factors and the interaction of them on falls and fall-related injuries. As the exposure to risk factors increases, the greater becomes the risk of falling and being injured.

a) Biological risk factors

Biological factors embrace characteristics of individuals that are pertaining to the human body. For instance, age, gender and race are non-modifiable biological factors. These are also associated with changes due to ageing such as the decline of physical, cognitive and affective capacities, and the co-morbidity associated with chronic illnesses.

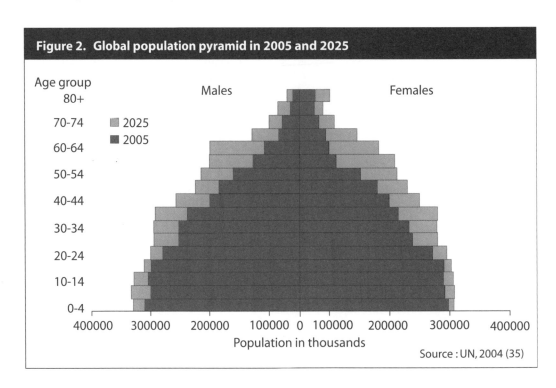

Figure 2. Global population pyramid in 2005 and 2025

Source : UN, 2004 (35)

Figure 3. Risk factor model for falls in older age

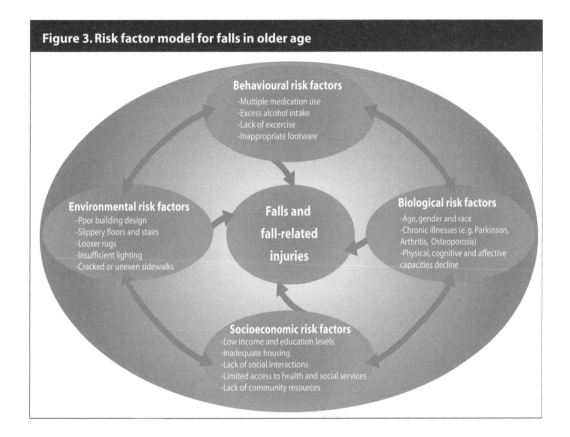

Behavioural risk factors
-Multiple medication use
-Excess alcohol intake
-Lack of excercise
-Inappropriate footware

Environmental risk factors
-Poor building design
-Slippery floors and stairs
-Looser rugs
-Insufficient lighting
-Cracked or uneven sidewalks

Falls and fall-related injuries

Biological risk factors
-Age, gender and race
-Chronic illnesses (e. g. Parkinson, Arthritis, Osteoporosis)
-Physical, cognitive and affective capacities decline

Socioeconomic risk factors
-Low income and education levels
-Inadequate housing
-Lack of social interactions
-Limited access to health and social services
-Lack of community resources

The interaction of biological factors with behavioural and environmental risks increases the risk of falling. For example, the loss of muscle strength leads to a loss of function and to a higher level of frailty, which intensifies the risk of falling due to some environmental hazards (see Chapter 3 for further information).

b) Behavioural risk factors

Behavioural risk factors include those concerning human actions, emotions or daily choices. They are potentially modifiable. For example, risky behaviour such as the intake of multiple medications, excess alcohol use, and sedentary behaviour can be modified through strategic interventions for behavioural change (see Chapter 3 and 4 for further information).

c) Environmental risk factors

Environmental factors encapsulate the interplay of individuals' physical conditions and the surrounding environment, including home hazards and hazardous features in public environment. These factors are not by themselves cause of falls – rather, the interaction between other factors and their exposure to environmental ones. Home hazards include narrow steps, slippery surfaces of stairs, looser rugs and insufficient lighting (29). Poor building design, slippery floor, cracked or uneven sidewalks, and poor lightening in public places are such hazards to injurious falls (see Chapter 3 for further information).

d) Socioeconomic risk factors

Socioeconomic risk factors are those related to influence social conditions and economic status of individuals as well as the capacity of the community to challenge them. These factors include: low income, low education, inadequate housing, lack of social interaction, limited access to health and social care especially in remote areas, and lack of community resources (see Chapter 3 for further information)

5. Main protective factors

Protective factors for falls in older age are related to behavioural change and environmental modification. Behavioural change to healthy lifestyle is a key ingredient to encourage healthy ageing and avoid falls. Non-smoking, moderate alcohol consumption, maintaining weight within normal range in mid to older age, playing an acceptable level of sport protect older people from falling (38). Furthermore, self-health behaviour (e.g. proper level of simple … walking) is integral to healthy ageing and independence.

One example of the environmental modifications is home modification. It prevents older persons from hidden fall hazards in daily activities at home. The modification includes installation of stairway protective devices such as railings, grab bars and slip-resistant surfacing in the bathroom and provision of lighting and handrails (39). Age-friendly design in public environment is also critical factor to avoid falls among older adults. (see Chapter 5 for further information).

6. Costs of falls

The economic impact of falls is critical to family, community, and society. Health-care impacts and costs of falls in older age are significantly increasing all over the world. Fall-incurred costs are categorized into two aspects:

Direct costs encompass health care costs such as medications and adequate services e.g. health-care-provider consultations in treatment and rehabilitation.

Indirect costs are societal productivity losses of activities in which individuals or family care givers would have involved if he/she had not sustain fall-related injuries e.g. lost income.

This section briefly shows an overview of health service impacts and costs of falls in some developed countries. This is due to the lack of data in developing countries.

a) Direct health system costs

The average health system cost per one fall injury episode for people 65 year and older in Finland and Australia was US$ 3611 (originally AUS$ 6500 in 2001-2002) and US$ 1049 (originally in €944 in 1999) respectively (23, 40).

Among different cost items, hospital inpatient services cost is the greatest cost, accounting for about 50% of total cost of falls (19, 22, 23). The cost of hospital inpatient services includes the emergency and general holding ward cost, of those admitted to either the general holding ward or to hospital. The second highest is the long-term care costs, contributing to 9.4% to 41% of all health system costs (23, 25).

The average cost of hospitalization for fall related injury for people 65 year and older range from US$ 6646 in Ireland to US$ 17 483 in the USA (22, 41). This cost are projected to increase to US$ 240 billion by year 2040 (42). Where the cost of a visit to an emergency department varies widely across countries, ranging from US$ 236 in the USA (based on data collected in 1998) (22) to US$ 2472 in Western Australia (based on data collected in 2001-2002) (23).

b) Indirect costs

In addition to the substantial direct costs outlined above, falls incur indirect costs that are critical to family e.g. the loss of productivity of family caregivers. The average lost earnings could approximate US$ 40 000 per annum in the United Kingdom (25). Even when family caregivers are more morally and culturally accepted, falls remain a significant burden to household economy.

7. References

1. Zecevic AA et al. (2006). Defining a fall and reasons for falling: Comparisons among the views of seniors, health care providers, and the research literature. *The Gerontologist*, 46:367-376.

2. Blake A et al.(1988). Falls by elderly people at home: prevalence and associated factors. Age Ageing, 17:365-372.

3. Prudham D, Evans J (1981). Factors associated with falls in the elderly: a community study. *Age Ageing*, 10:141-146.

4. Campbell AJ et al. (1981). Falls in old age: a study of frequency and related clinical factors. *Age Ageing*, 10:264-270.

5. Tinetti ME, Speechley M, Ginter SF (1988). Risk factors for falls among elderly persons living in the   community. *New England Journal of Medicine*, 319:1701-1707.

6. Downton JH, Andrews K (1991). Prevalence, characteristics and factors associated with falls among the elderly living at home. *Aging* (Milano), 3(3):219-28.

7. Stalenhoef PA et al. (2002). A risk model for the prediction of recurrent falls in community-dwelling elderly: A prospective cohort study. *Journal of Clinical Epidemiology*, 55(11):1088-1094.

8. Tinetti ME (1987). Factors associated with serious injury during falls by ambulatory nursing home residents. *Journal of the American Geriatrics Society*, 35:644-648.

9. Wannian Liang, Ying Liu, e.a. Xueqing Weng (2004). An epidemiological study on injury of the community-dwelling elderly in Beijing. *Chinese Journal of Disease Control and Prevention*, 8(6):489-492.

10. Suzhen L, Jiping L, Y C (2004). Body function and fall-related factors of the elderly in community. *Journal of Nursing Science*, 19(6):5-7.

11. Weiping M, Lihua Y (2002). Analysis of risk factors for elderly falls. *Chinese Journal of Behavioural Medical Science*, 11(6):697-699.

12. Gang L, Sufang J, YS (2006). The incidence status on injury of the community-dwelling elderly in Beijing (in Chinese). *Chinese Journal of Preventive Medicine*, 40(1):37.

13. Litao L, Shengyong W, Shong Y (2002). A study on risk factors for falling down in elderly people of rural areas in Laizhou city. *Chinese Journal of Geriatrics*, 21(5):370-372.

14. Yoshida H, Kim H (2006). Frequency of falls and their prevention (in Japanese). *Clinical Calcium*, 16(9):1444-1450.

15. Reyes-Ortiz CA, Al Snih S, Markides KS (2005). Falls among elderly persons in Latin America and the Caribbean and among elderly Mexican-Americans. *Revista Panamericana de Salud Pública*, 17(5-6):362-369.

16. Stevens JA, Sogolow ED (2005). Gender differences for non-fatal unintentional fall related injuries among older adults. *Injury Prevention*, 11(2):115-119.

17. Gregg EW et al. (2000). Diabetes and physical disability among older U.S. adults. *Diabetes Care*, 23(9):1272-1277.

18. Scuffham P, Chaplin S, Legood R (2003). Incidence and costs of unintentional falls in older people in the United Kingdom. *Journal of Epidemiology and Community Health*, 57:740-744.

19. Scott VJ (2005). Technical report: hospitalizations due to falls among Canadians age 65 and over. In Report on Seniors' falls in Canada. Canada, Minister of Public Works and Government Services.

20. Seematter-Bagnoud L et al. (2006). Healthcare utilization of elderly persons hospitalized after a noninjurious fall in a Swiss academic medical center. *Journal of the American Geriatrics Society*, 4(6):891-897.

21. Bergeron E et al. (2006). A simple fall in the elderly: not so simple. *Journal of Trauma*, 60(2):268-273.

22. Roudsari B et al. (2005). The acute medical care costs of fall-related injuries among the U.S. older adults. Injury, 36(11):1316-1322.

23. Hendrie D et al. (2003). Injury in Western Australia: The health system costs of falls in older adults in Western Australia. Perth, Western Australia, Western Australian Government.

24. Herman M, Gallagher E, Scott VJ (2006). The evolution of seniors' falls prevention in British Columbia. Victoria, British Colombia, British Columbia Ministry of Health http://www.health.gov.bc.ca/library/publications/year/2006/falls_report.pdf, accessed 27 August 2007).

25. The University of York (2000). The economic cost of hip fracture in the U.K., *Health Promotion*, England.

26. Zuckerman JD (1996). Hip fracture. *New England Journal of Medicine*, 334(23):1519-1525.

27. Rubenstein LZ (2006). Falls in older people: epidemiology, risk factors and strategies for prevention. *Age Ageing*, 35-S2:ii37-ii41.

28. Stevens JA et al. (2007). Fatalities and Injuries From Falls Among Older Adults, United States, 1993-2003 and 2001-2005. *Journal of the American Medical Association*, 297(1):32-33.

29. Division of Aging and Seniors, PHAC. Canada (2005). Report on senior's fall in Canada. Ontario, Division of Aging and Seniors. Public Health Agency of Canada.

30. Kannus P et al (2005). Fall-induced deaths among elderly people. *American Public Health Association*, 95(3):422-424.

31. National Council on Ageing (2005). Falls among older adults: risk factors and prevention strategies. In Fall free: promoting a national falls prevention action plan. J.A. Stevens Eds..

32. Fransen M et al. (2002). Excess mortality or institutionalization after hip fracture: men are at greater risk than women. *Journal of the American Geriatrics Society*, 50(4):685-690.

33. Hernandez JL et al. (2006). Trend in hip fracture epidemiology over a 14-year period in a Spanish population. *Osteoporosis International*, 17: 464-470.

34. World Health Organization (2002). Active Ageing: A Policy Framework. Geneva.

35. United Nations (UN) (2004). World Population Prospects: The 2004 Revision. New York, USA.

36. Kannus P et al. (2007). Alarming rise in the number and incidence of fall-induced cervical spine injuries among older adults. *Journal of Gerontology*: Biological Sciences and Medical Sciences, 62(2):180-183.

37. Kalache A, Keller I (2000). The greying world: a challenge for the 21st century. *Science Progress*, 83(1):33-54.

38. Peel NM, McClure RJ, Hendrikz JK (2006). Health-protective behaviours and risk of fall-related hip fractures: a population-based case-control study. doi: 10.1093/ageing/afl056. Age Ageing, 35(5):491-497.

39. American Geriatrics Society, British Geriatrics Society, and American Academy of Orthopaedic Surgeons Panel on Falls Prevention (2001). Guideline for the prevention of falls in older persons. *Journal of the American Geriatrics Society*, 49(5):664-672.

40. Nurmi I., Luthje P (2002). Incidence and costs of falls and fall injuries among elderly in institutional care. *Scandinavian Journal of Primary Health Care*, 20(2):118-122.

41. Carey D, Laffoy M (2005). Hospitalisations due to falls in older persons. *Irish Medical Journal,* 98(6):179-181.

42. Cummings SR, Rubin SM, Black D (1990). The future of hip fractures in the United States. Numbers, costs, and potential effects of postmenopausal estrogen. Clinical Orthopaedics and Related Research, (252):163-166.

Chapter II. Active Ageing: a framework for the global strategy for the prevention of falls in older age

The WHO's Active Ageing policy offers a coherent framework on which to develop a strategy for the prevention of falls in older age worldwide.

a) What is 'Active Ageing'?

Active Ageing is the process of optimizing opportunities for health, participation and security in order to enhance quality of life as people age.

Active Ageing depends on a variety of influences or determinants that surround individuals, families and communities as expressed in Figure 1 below. They include gender and culture, which are cross-cutting, and six additional groups of complementary and interrelated determinants:

1. access to health and social services,

2. behavioural,

3. physical environment,

4. personal,

5. social, and

6. economic.

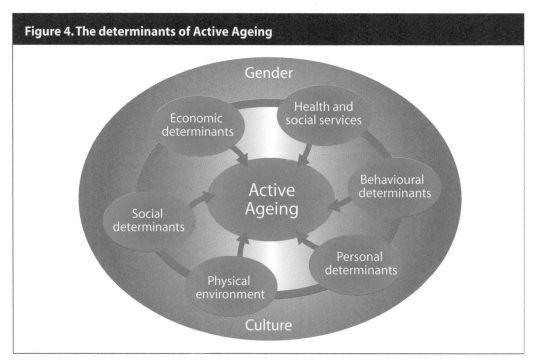

Figure 4. The determinants of Active Ageing

Source: *Active Ageing: A Policy Framework*, WHO, 2002 (http://www.who.int/ageing/publications/active/en/index.html)

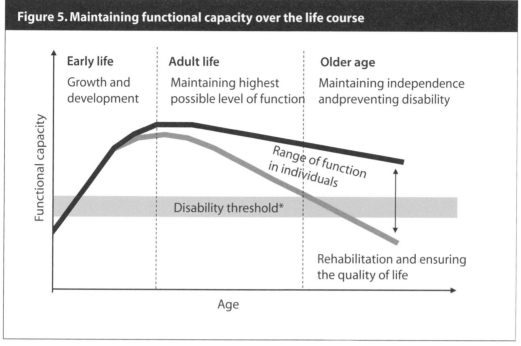

Figure 5. Maintaining functional capacity over the life course

Source: *Active Ageing: A Policy Framework*, WHO, 2002

In addition, there are the underlying 'biological' factors which can play a significant role as preventing individuals from falls and consequent injuries or, conversely, can act as risk factors. All of these determinants, and the interplay between them, play an important role in affecting how high or low is the risk of falling and/or if a fall occurs, the risk of sustaining serious injuries.

These determinants have to be understood from a life course perspective which recognizes that older persons are not a homogeneous group and that individual diversity increases with age. This is expressed in Figure 2 (next page), which illustrates that functional capacity (such as muscular strength and cardiovascular output) increases in childhood to peak in early adulthood and eventually decline. The rate

of decline is largely determined by factors related to lifestyle behaviours, as well as external social, environmental and economic factors. From an individual and societal perspective, it is important to remember that the speed of decline can be influenced and may be reversible at any age through individual and public policy measures, such as promoting an age-friendly living environment. An example of particular importance within the context of falls, relates to bone mass. Good nutrition and optimum levels of physical activity throughout childhood and adolescence are critical for the development of healthy bones. As individuals age they experience a gradual decline in bone mass. Once again, healthy life styles can slow down the process. For post menopausal women in particular, such life styles are crucially important to counterbalance the hormonal factors that can precipitate the onset of osteoporosis. For some secondary prevention through drug-therapy becomes an indispensable form of intervention for avoiding bone fractures as a consequence of even relatively minor traumas.

Active ageing is a lifelong process. Thus, age-friendly environments with barrier-free buildings and streets, adequate public transportation and accessible sources of information and communication enhance the mobility and independence of younger as well as older persons who present the risk of developing disabilities. Secure neighbourhoods allow children, younger women and older persons to venture outside in confidence to participate in physically active leisure and in social activities – contributing to preventing falls at all ages, particularly at old age. The operative word in a society committed to active ageing is enablement – for instance through initiatives such as:

- Affordable parking is available.

- Priority parking bays are provided for older people close to buildings and transport stops.

- Priority parking bays are provided for people with disabilities close to buildings and transport stops, the use of which are monitored.

- Drop off and pick up bays close to buildings and transport stops are provided for handicapped and older people.

2. References

1. World Health Organization. Active Ageing – A Policy Framework. Geneva: World Health Organization, 2002.

Chapter III. Determinants of Active Ageing as they relate to falls in older age

Approaching falls in older age within the framework of the determinants of Active Ageing help us to develop effective interventions and policies. The following section summarizes what is known about how the determinants of Active Ageing affect falls in older age.

1. Cross-cutting determinants: culture and gender

a) Culture

> Cultural values and traditions determine to a large extent how a given society views older people and falls in older age.

Culturally driven expectations affect how people view older persons and falls in older age. In some cultures, social participation in older age is not seen as a virtue: the perception is that old people are meant "to rest". In practice, this results in some older people adopting sedentary life often in isolation due to the resignation from social, economic and cultural participation, with a resulting increase in the risk of falling. Furthermore, in many societies, falls in older age are perceived as "an inevitable natural part of ageing" or "unavoidable accidents". All these contribute to falls prevention not to be considered as a matter of priority on governmental agendas - leading to a loss of financial provisions required to develop surveillance systems, appropriate interventions and clinical diagnostic techniques, as well as treatment regimens for falls and fall-related injuries.

Cultural preferences are also reflected in the design of public and private spaces – such as shining floors and steps or staircases without appropriate railings.

Culture also contributes to the stigma of requesting help where that is needed or even unavoidable – for instance, where negotiating architectonic barriers that should not be there in the first place but, if they are, asking for help should come naturally rather than a reason for embarrassment.

b) Gender

> While falls are more common among older women than men fall-related mortality is higher among older men. Policies and programmes on falls prevention need to reflect a gender perspective.

As is outlined in Chapter 1, women are more likely than men to fall and sustain fracture (1), resulting in twice more hospitalizations and emergency department visits than men (2). However, fall-related mortality disproportionately affects men.

The difference in falls in older age may stem from the gender-related factors, such as women being inclined to make greater use of multiple medications and living alone (3). In addition, biological difference also contributes to greater risk, for instance, women's muscle mass declines faster than that of men, especially in the immediate few years after menopause. To some extent this is gender-related as women are less likely to engage into the practice of muscular building physical activity though the life course e.g. sports.

Health seeking behaviour differs according to gender. Culturally-oriented expectations to gender roles affect behaviour when seeking medical care. Male higher fatality rates may be due in part to the tendency of men not seeking medical care until a condition becomes severe, resulting in substantial delay to the access to prevention and management of diseases. Further, men are more likely to be engaged in intense and dangerous physical activity and risky behaviours – such as climbing high ladders, cleaning roofs or ignoring the limits of their physical capacity.

Various policy options and falls prevention strategies for men and women based on gender differences in locations, circumstances and events preceding falls and fall-related injuries are needed.

2. Determinants related to health and social services

Health and social services providers are by and large unprepared to prevent and manage falls in older age.

Falls in older age has been a neglected public health problem in many societies, particularly in the developing world. Many health and social services providers are unprepared to prevent and manage falls in older age as they lack sufficient knowledge to treat the conditions that predispose their consequences and complications.

Falls in older age are often iatrogenic conditions – that is, induced by incorrect diagnoses and treatments. Examples include over-prescription of medications that cause side effects and interactions among the drugs, inadequate dosage and lack of warning to make older people aware about their effects.

Appropriate training programmes covering knowledge and skills in falls prevention and management should be a priority in primary heath care (PHC) settings, where increasing number of patients are older people. PHC practitioners should be well versed in the diagnosis and management of falls and fall-related injuries. In addition, social services that ensure the accessibility of older people to falls prevention programmes are critical.

3. Behavioural determinants

a) Physical activity

> Regular participation in moderate physical activity is integral to good health and maintaining independence, contributing to lowering risk of falls and fall-related injuries.

Regular participation in moderate physical activity is integral to good health and maintaining independence. It prevents onset of multiple pathologies and functional capacity decline. Moderate physical activities and exercise also lowers risk of falls and fall-related injuries in older age through controlling weight as well as contributing to healthy bones, muscles, and joints (4). Exercise can improve balance, mobility and reaction time. It can increases bone mineral density of postmenopausal women and individuals aged 70 years and over (5).

Moreover, it should be noticed that participation in vigorous physical activities – for instance intensive running in older age may increase the risk of falls. Promoting appropriate physical activities or exercises to improve strength, balance, and flexibility is one of the most feasible and cost-effective strategies to prevent falls among older adults in the community. Activities such as outdoor walking or mall walking indoors is the most feasible and accessible way of exercising that improves strength, balance and flexibility leading to a reduction on the risk of falling. Other kind of effective physical activities and exercises are mentioned in Chapter 5.

b) Healthy eating

> Eating a balanced diet rich in calcium may decrease the risk injuries resulting from falls in older people.

Eating a healthy balanced diet is central to healthy ageing. Adequate intake of protein, calcium, essential vitamins and water are essential for optimum health. If deficiencies do exist, it is reasonable to expect that weakness, poor fall recovery and increase risk of injuries will ensure. Growing evidence supports dietary calcium and vitamin D intake improves bone mass among persons with low bone density and that it reduces the risk of osteoporosis and falling (6). No dairy and fish consumption were associated with a higher risk of falling. Older persons with low dietary intake of calcium and vitamin D may be at risk for falls and therefore fractures resulting from them (7).

Use of excessive alcohol has been shown to be a risk factor of falls. Consumption of 14 or more drinks per week is associated with an increased risk of falls in older adults (7).

c) Use of medicines

Older people tend to take more drugs than younger people. Also as people age, they develop altered mechanisms for absorbing and metabolizing drugs. If older persons don't take medications as directed by health professionals, their risk of falling can be affected in several ways. Effects of uncontrolled medical conditions and of medication because of non-adherence can provoke or generate altering alertness, judgement, and coordination; dizziness; altering the balance mechanism and the ability to recognize and adapt to obstacles; and increased stiffness or weakness (7).

When prescribing new drugs to these older patients health professionals should fully ascertain other drugs being taken, including self-prescribed medicines.

d) Risk-taking behaviours

> The ordinary choices people make and the actions they take may increase their chance of falling.

Some risk-taking behaviours increase the risk of falling in older age. Those behaviours include climbing ladders, standing on unsteady chairs or bending while performing activities of daily living, rushing with little attention to the environment or not using mobility devices prescribed to them such as a cane or walker (8).

Wearing poor fitting shoes is also a risk taking behaviour. Walking in socks without shoes or in slippers without a sole increases the risk of slipping indoor. Appropriate shoes are particularly important – avoiding high heels, thin and hard soles, or slippers of unsuitable size and that do not stick closely to the feet.

4. Determinants related to personal factors

a) Attitudes

> People's attitudes influence their behaviours. Attitudes affect how people interpret and cope with falls in older age.

Older people's attitudes greatly influence whether they will avoid fall-related risk-taking behaviours when they participate in activities of daily living. If older people perceive falls as a normal consequence of ageing expressed as "seniors will always fall" their attitudes may halt preventive measures.

Attitudes of policy-makers determine to a large extent the amount of resources allocated to falls prevention and development and enforcement of related policies. Awareness and attitudes of health professionals to falls are essential to increased incentive in providing appropriate services for preventing and managing falls in older age.

Professionals who design public transportations, such as buses and subway systems, often do not make them age-friendly, neglecting the risk of falls for older people. For example, in some developing countries, buses are designed with not enough seats and rails and the steps to climb into them are too high. As a consequence, older people incur the risk of falling because they have to stand or do not have the strength to climb into the buses in the first place and cannot properly hold on for support. Moreover, the steps on the public buses are often too high to older people and they might fall when getting into the bus.

b) Fear of falling

Fear of falling is frequently reported by older persons. Older people are usually under the fear of falling again, being hurt or hospitalized, not being able to get up after a fall, social embarrassment, loss of independence, and having to move from their homes. Fear can positively motivate some seniors to take precautions against falls and can lead to gait adaptations that increase stability. For others, fear can lead to a decline in overall quality of life and increase the risk of falls through a reduction in the activities needed to maintain self-esteem, confidence, strength and balance. In addition, fear can lead to maladaptive changes in balance control that may increase the risk of falling. People who are fearful of falling also tend to lack confidence in their ability to prevent or manage falls, which increases the risk of falling again (7).

c) Coping with falls

The ability of coping with falls of both older people and health professionals can lower the risk and consequences of falling.

Falls are particularly difficult to manage in PHC settings because health professionals lack enough knowledge and skills. Building coping skills of health professionals to prevent and manage falls needs to be emphasized. For example, health professionals are recommended to teach patients at risk of falling how to get up from the floor; unfortunately clinical experience suggests that this is rarely done (9).

Physical and mental management of falls by older people and their family members is also important. Therefore, training older people at high risk to avoid falling needs to be encouraged.

d) Ethnicity and race

Although the relationship between falls and ethnicity and race remains widely open for research, Caucasians living in the USA have higher risk of falling. In addition, for both men and women, the rate of hospitalization for fall-related injuries is some two to four times higher among the Whites than Hispanics and Asians/Pacific Islanders, and about 20% higher than African-Americans (10). It is also clear differences observed between Singaporeans of Chinese, Malay and Indian ethnic origins, and between native Japanese older community dwellers and Japanese-Americans and Caucasians. Native Japanese people have much lower rates of falls than Japanese-Americans and Caucasians.

5. Determinants related to the physical environment

> Factors related to the physical environment are the most common cause of falls in older age.

Physical environment plays a significant role in many falls in older age. Factors related to the physical environment are the most common cause of falls in older people, responsible for between 30 to 50% of them (11). A number of hazards in the home and public environment that interact with other risk factors, such as poor vision or balance, contribute to falls and fall-related injuries. For example, stairs can be problematic – studies show that unsafe features of stairs can be frequently identified including uneven or excessively high or narrow steps, slippery surfaces, unmarked edges, discontinuous or poorly-fitted handrails, and inadequate or excessive lighting.

Since approximately half of falls occurs indoor, the home environment is critical for avoiding them. A high particular risk to falls was found in homes with irregular sidewalks to the residence, loose carpets on the kitchen and bathroom floors, loose electrical wires, and inconvenient doorsteps. Poor surroundings around home such as garden paths and walks that are cracked or slippery from rain, snow or moss are also dangerous. Entrance stairs and poor night lighting can also pose risks.

Factors related to the public environment are also frequent causes of fall in older age. Even walking on a familiar route can lead to falls as a consequence of poor building design and inadequate consideration. Most problematic factors are cracked or uneven sidewalks, unmarked obstacles, slippery surfaces, poor lighting and lengthy distances to sitting areas and public restrooms.

6. Determinants related to the social environment

> Social connection and inclusion are vital to health in older age. Social interaction is inversely related to the risk of falls.

Isolation and loneliness are commonly experiences by older people particularly among those who lose their spouse or live alone. They are much more likely than other groups to experience disability and the physical, cognitive, and sensory limitations that increase the risk of falls.

Isolation and depression triggered by lack of social participation increase fear of falling, and vice versa. Fear of falling can increase the risk of falls through a reduction in social participation and loss of personal contact - which in turn increase isolation and depression. Providing social support and opportunities for older people to participate in social activities to help maintain active interaction with others may decrease their risk of falls.

7. Economic determinants

> Older people with lower economic status, especially those who are female, live alone or in rural areas face an increased risk of falls.

Studies have shown that there is a relationship between socioeconomic status and falls. Lower income is associated with increased risk of falling (12). Older people, especially those who are female, live alone or in rural areas with unreliable and insufficient incomes face an increased risk of falls. Poor environment in which they live, their poor diet and the fact of not being able to access health care services even when they have acute or chronic illness exacerbates the risk of falling.

The negative cycle of poverty and falls in older age is particularly evident in rural areas and in developing countries. The fall-related burden to health system will keep increasing unless resources and money are allocated in order to provide proper PHC and opportunities to older people for social participation. It is never too late to break this vicious cycle.

8. References

1. Stevens JA et al. (2006). The costs of fatal and non-fatal falls among older adults. *Injury Prevention*, 12(5):290-295.

2. Hendrie D et al. (2003). Injury in Western Australia: The Health System Cost of Falls in Older Adults in Western Australia. Perth, Western Australia. Western Australian Government.

3. Ebrahim S, Kalache A (1996). Epidemiology in Old Age. London, Blackwell *BMJ* Books.

4. Gardner MM, Robertson MG, Campbell AJ (2000). Exercise in preventing falls and fall related injuries in older people: A review of randomised controlled trials. *British Journal of Sports Medicine*, 34:7-17.

5. Day M et al. (2002). Randomised factorial trial of falls prevention among older people living in their own homes. *BMJ*, doi:10.1136/bmj.325.7356.128.

6. Tuck SP, Francis RM (2002). Osteoporosis. *Postgraduate Medical Journal*, 78:526-532.

7. Division of Aging and Seniors (2005). Report on senior's fall in Canada. Ontario. Public Health Agency of Canada.

8. Gallagher EH, Brunt H (1996). Head over heels: A clinical trial to reduce falls among the elderly. *Canadian Journal on Aging*, 15:84-96.

9. Simpson JM, Salkin S (1993). Are elderly people at risk of falling taught how to get up again? Age Ageing, 22: 294-296.

10. Ellis AA, Trent RB (2001). Hospitalized fall injuries and race in California. *Injury Prevention*, 7:316-320.

11. Rubenstein LZ (2006). Falls in older people: epidemiology, risk factors and strategies for prevention. *Age and Ageing*, 35-S2:ii37-ii41.

12. Reyes CA et al. (2004). Risk factors for falling in older Mexican Americans. *Ethnicity & Disease*, 14:417-422.

Chapter IV. Challenges for prevention of falls in older age

1. Changing behaviour to prevent falls

The background papers that underlie this report refer to a considerable body of evidence indicating the effectiveness of a number of interventions for falls prevention. These include strength and balance training, environmental modification and medical care aimed at removing or reducing specific risk factors by for example review of medications and reduction of polypharmacy. The systematic reviews, evidence syntheses and meta-analyses are well referenced in the briefing papers to be found at the following WHO URL:

http://www.who.int/ageing/projects/falls_prevention_older_age/en/index.html

Crucial to the success of such interventions is changing the beliefs, attitudes and behaviour of older people themselves, the health and social care professionals who provide services, and the wider communities in which older people live. For example, a fifteen-week balance and exercise class will only have an effect if the older person goes to the sessions, undertakes the exercises as prescribed, and continues to practice after completion of the course. People will only change their lifestyles if:

- it is within their ability to do so;

- they have the resources to implement change (including physical, psychological and social capital resources);

- the changes are perceived as being of benefit to them; and

- the benefit outweighs the cost or effort in overcoming barriers.

For example, the older person may care for grandchildren, and thus using time to do exercises to maintain or improve physical function may appear in the immediate term a poor use of time or impossible if it conflicts with childcare responsibilities. Thus, the programme will need to be tailored to fit with these responsibilities, or the person must be persuaded that a long-term gain (maintaining independence and seeing the grandchildren grow up) outweighs the short-term 'pain'. Most importantly, the society in which older people live must value them and be willing to allocate resources to the maintenance of their health and well-being. Expression of valuing older people must include allocation of adequate resources towards helping people to age well and take part in activities that have the potential to prevent falls.

This chapter is based heavily on a series of recommendations made by the Psychological Aspects of Falling Group (1, 2), Work Package 4 of the Prevention of Falls Network Europe (ProFaNE) and fuller evidence for the recommendations has been published (1, 2). These recommendations should be sufficiently general to be applicable to populations other than the European population for which they were originally developed.

a) Raise awareness in the general population of a number of interventions that could improve balance and prevent falls.

To make choices people need to have at least basic information about benefits of taking part in activities aimed at prevention. But information alone is not enough, it needs to be framed so that it promotes realistic positive beliefs about the possibilities for preventive action if any change is likely to follow. Many older people seem to assume that falls prevention consists of activity restriction or the use of aids and home modifications. Research suggests that many older people are ignorant that fall risks can be reduced because there is a fatalistic acceptance of falling that may contribute to low uptake of falls prevention interventions.

Campaigns need to raise general awareness and should not be aimed only at older people. The opinions of others, including health professionals and family, influence older people's decisions.

At present, advice from family members and health professionals tends to emphasize avoiding risk rather than engaging in activities to improve strength and balance (3-5). Informing the general population about the benefits of easy-to-provide interventions such as strength and balance training activities should influence older people's views and counteract fatalistic views that falling is a consequence of ageing (6). Exercise may be generally recognized as important for maintaining fitness and strength, but its importance in maintaining good balance and function needs to be better publicized. It is likely that the approach will prove effective for both high and lower-risk populations (7). Although the effectiveness of less intensive interventions at a population level is currently unknown it would seem likely that they will provide benefit. Exercises that improve strength and balance should be recommended for all older people (7-9).

Emphasis must be on the positive advantages of undertaking interventions such as balance and exercise training, rather than on reduction of risk of falls since the latter is generally viewed negatively and of little relevance by many older people. Uptake may be encouraged by promoting greater awareness among older people, their families and health professionals of how undertaking specific physical activities may contribute to improving balance and reducing falls risk.

b) When offering or publicizing interventions, promote benefits that fit with a positive self-identity.

It seems that many older people do not acknowledge falls, for example because of fear of:

- negative stereotyping;

- beliefs that falls are an inevitable and unavoidable consequence of ageing; and

- embarrassment about loss of control.

Falls prevention advice is often perceived as being for other 'disabled or elderly people'. Programmes that are perceived to impact negatively on self-image are likely to be unattractive while those, which are viewed as improving skills or characteristics valued by older people, are likely to be more popular. In interviews older people say that they would participate in falls-prevention initiatives to be proactive in managing their own health needs, maintain independence and improve confidence (4, 5). Older people value strength and balance training activities for their potential to:

- maintain functional capabilities and thus avoid disability and dependence;

- enhance general health, mobility and appearance; and

- be interesting, enjoyable and sociable (4, 5).

These characteristics are all compatible with a positive identity and should be encouraged.

Uptake of falls prevention interventions may be enhanced by emphasizing the positive benefits that are likely to accord with desirable self images for older people, in addition to those that reduce fall risks. Examples of such benefits include increased independence, greater confidence, ability to take an active part in society and support younger generations.

c) Utilize a variety of forms of social encouragement to engage older people

Uptake may be encouraged by the use of personal invitations to participate (from a health professional or other authority figures) and positive media images and peer role models to illustrate the social acceptability, safety and multiple benefits of taking part. Uptake and adherence may be encouraged by ongoing support from family, peers, professionals and social organizations. A wide range of social influences are known to impact on health-related behaviour, including encouragement, approval and social support from health professionals and other sources (10). Role models should provide examples of successful accomplishment of health-related goals (11). Concern about social disapproval poses a barrier to undertaking physical activity, while social support, positive media images and real-life examples of ordinary older people doing exercise can promote greater physical activity (12-14).

Social factors play a key role in people's decisions whether to participate in falls prevention interventions (15, 16). In European countries a personal invitation from a trusted health professional is an important motivation for taking up an intervention, and approval and encouragement from family, friends and health professionals influence initial and continued participation (5). Participation in group activities is influenced by anticipated and actual positive and negative social contacts with members and leaders of the group. A major barrier is the perception that falls prevention is only for very old and frail people and not relevant to oneself (3-5). Inversely, old and frail people may see health promoting activities as strenuous and only suitable for people who are younger and fitter (6). Since seeing prevention activities as appropriate for someone like oneself is the foremost predictor of intention to undertake these activities (3, 17) it may be valuable to use media pictures and peer role models to promote a positive social image of strength and balance training. The latter is as a suitable activity for those who are still fit and active, in order to maintain their mobility and independence, while emphasizing that it can still be a safe and effective method of falls prevention for those at higher risk of falling.

d) Ensure that the intervention is designed to meet the needs, preferences and capabilities of the individual.

Review of evidence generally suggests that a tailored personal approach – even for group contexts – can greatly improve the chance of older people engaging with and maintaining an intervention programme (1-2). There is a need to consider the individual's lifestyle, values, religious and cultural beliefs, which may be associated with ethnicity and gender-specific factors. Environmental determinants such as the wealth of the society in which the older person lives; their place of residence and availability and access to services should also be contemplated. Interventions need to be presented in ways that are tailored to the cultural preferences of older people and be realistic within the resources available. Group sessions with trained-balance and strength-exercise instructors for example, are relatively low-tech affordable interventions that should be within the means of many societies. Although more research is necessary, there is growing evidence that many older people may prefer exercises delivered at home with some professional guidance (4, 12).

Cost-effective ways of catering for these preferences at a public health level should be considered when developing a policy. The evidence-based principles of balance and strength training could be presented as part of a set of activities that are recognizable and accepted within specific cultures. For example, while exercises, which promote physical strength and balance, may be presented within T'ai Chi Ch'uan based practice appropriately in China, a more suitable presentation of exercises, which promote physical strength and balance in India, may be based on yogic practices. Dance may provide a vehicle for adequate exercises in a number of cultures. How exercises are best presented will need to be developed locally and should be tested before large-scale roll out of a programme in a country.

e) Encourage self-management rather than dependence on professionals by giving older people an active role.

There is strong theoretical rationale in the psychology literature generally to suggest that participation and adherence will be maximized if the older person can choose or modify the intervention (1-2). While some form of supervision will be necessary to ensure safety and appropriate components, the older person should be enabled, wherever possible, to select among:

- different interventions;

- different formats of the same intervention; or

- a range of intervention goals.

f) Draw on validated methods for promoting and assessing the processes that maintain adherence, especially in the longer term.

These could include encouraging realistic positive beliefs, assisting with planning and implementation of new behaviours, building self-confidence, and providing practical support. There is substantial evidence for a range of techniques for changing health-related behaviour but it is most effective to combine a variety of such approaches (10). Potentially important ingredients include:

- creating a supportive partnership relationship with the therapy provider (see recommendations 3 and 5);

- providing with good practical support (access and appropriate supervision);

- promoting the belief that the intervention is necessary and effective;

- building confidence in being able to carry out the intervention;

- developing skills for generating and maintaining new behaviours (e.g. goal-setting, planning, self-monitoring, and self-reward); and

- tailoring interventions to individual needs (see recommendation 4).

2. References

1. Yardley L et al. Recommendations for promoting the engagement of older people in preventive health care. Manchester, ProFaNE, Workpackage 4 (http://www.profane.eu.org/directory/display_resource.php?resource_id=1121, accessed 27 August 2007).

2. Yardley L et al. (2007). Recommendations for promoting the engagement of older people in activities to prevent falls. *Quality and Safety in Health Care*, 16(3):230-234.

3. Yardley L, Todd C. (2005). Encouraging positive attitudes to falls in later life. London, Help the Aged.

4. Yardley L et al. (2006). Older people's views of advice about falls prevention: a qualitative study. *Health Education Research*, 21:508-517.

5. Yardley L et al. (2006). Older people's views of falls-prevention interventions in six European countries. *The Gerontologist*, 46:650-660.

6. Simpson JM, Darwin C, Marsh N (2003). What are older people prepared to do to avoid falling? A qualitative study in London. *British Journal of Community Nursing*, 8:152-159.

7. Chang JT et al. (2004). Interventions for the prevention of falls in older adults: systematic review and meta-analysis of randomised clinical trials. *British Medical Journal*, 328:680-683.

8. Kannus P et al. (2005). Prevention of falls and consequent injuries in elderly people. *Lancet*, 366:1885-1893.

9. Skelton D, Todd C (2004). What are the main risk factors for falls amongst older people and what are the most effective interventions to prevent these falls? Copenhagen, WHO Regional Office for Europe, Health Evidence Network report, (http://www.euro.who.int/document/E82552.pdf, accessed 27 August 2007).

10. World Health Organization (2003). Adherence to long-term therapies: evidence for action. Geneva.

11. Bandura A (1997). Self-efficacy: the exercise of control. New York, WH Freeman.

12. King AC et al. (2000). Personal and environmental factors associated with physical inactivity among different racial-ethnic groups of US middle-aged and older-aged women. *Health Psychology*, 19:354-364.

13. King AC, Rejeski WJ, Buchner DM (1998). Physical activity interventions targeting older adults: A critical review and recommendations. *American Journal of Preventive Medicine*, 15:316-333.

14. Ory M et al. (2003). Challenging aging stereotypes: strategies for creating a more active society. *American Journal of Preventive Medicine*, 25:164-171.

15. Commonwealth Department of Health and Aged Care (2001). National Falls Prevention for Older People Initiative "Step out with confidence". Canberra, Commonwealth of Australia.

16. McInnes E, Askie L (2004). Evidence review on older people's views and experiences of falls prevention strategies. *Worldviews on Evidence-Based Nursing*, 1:20-37.

17. Yardley L et al. (2007). Attitudes and beliefs that predict older people's intention to undertake strength and balance training. *Journals of Gerontology Series B, Psychological Sciences and Social Sciences*, 62B:119-125.

Chapter V. Examples of effective policies and interventions

As discussed in previous sections, the effect of a fall on an older person can be a devastating event, resulting in chronic pain, loss of independence and a reduced quality of life. Moreover, the cumulative effect of falls and resulting injuries among older persons in most countries has the potential to reach epidemic proportions that would consume a disproportionate amount of health care resources. Healthy public policies and proven prevention strategies are needed to provide the infrastructure and support essential for the integration of fall prevention evidence into practice. The complex and multifactorial nature of fall risk among a rapidly ageing and growing population demands a proactive and systematic approach to prevention that integrates policy, preventive measures and practice.

- Policy should provide the infrastructure and support essential to a comprehensive and integrated approach to falls prevention.

- Prevention evidence is needed to support the effective application of proven interventions.

- Practice is where evidence is applied accordingly to the standards and protocols set by policy.

1. Policy

To effectively address the growing problem of falls in an ageing society, healthy public policies are needed to provide vision, set priorities and establish institutional standards. Such policies should facilitate capacity building unique to each setting by supporting the generation of new research, encouraging broad collaboration and maximizing availability of resources.

Falls and resulting injuries among older persons are public health problems in all regions of the world that are facing the impact of an ageing population. The good news is that evidence exists to show that most falls are both predicable and preventable. There are also good examples to show that this evidence can be applied to sustainable changes in practice when supported by healthy public policies. Examples of such policies are more commonly seen in developed countries where healthy public policies have established capacity for effective falls prevention through good leadership, intersectoral collaboration and education. Moreover, these are the countries that have first experienced population ageing and have had the necessary financial resources to implement such policies.

a) Leadership

Government agencies responsible for health and social services for older persons are well placed to provide leadership by establishing a policy-making infrastructure, collaborating to set priorities and targets, and overseeing and supporting national and regional efforts to reduce falls and related injuries.

community-service providers, researchers, community planners, policy-makers and many other potential partners for creating integrated falls prevention activities. Strategies for developing and maintaining collaboration include the formation of focused fall-prevention coalitions.

Many recommendations from the Falls Free Coalition National Action Plan are now

Leadership

An example of such leadership is seen in Canada, where a turning point in policy development for falls prevention occurred in 1999 when a policy-maker in the Province of British Columbia (B.C.) Ministry of Health, set in place a collaborative process for priority setting to reduce falls and fall-related injury rates for the province. The process involved an analysis of regional data on the scope and nature of the problem combined with meetings of regional stakeholders to identify priority areas for change. The final product was a comprehensive report of fall-related morbidity and mortality, a review of the literature on fall-risk factors and proven prevention strategies, and 31 priority recommendations for policy and prevention (1, 2). The process of meaningful involvement by the stakeholders in the formation of these recommendations was pivotal to the success of this leadership model. Since release of this report, there has been substantial growth in the number of falls prevention programmes and a significant reduction in fall-related deaths and hospitalizations among older persons in B.C. (3).

b) Collaboration

A good leader will recognize that the most important collaborators in developing effective falls prevention policies are those most directly impacted by the issue – older persons at risk of falling, those who care for them, and those who provide services to older adults. This comprehensive approach serves to include health-care providers,

included in a recently passed USA Senate Committee Falls Prevention Bill, with US$ 8 million of authorized spending for fall-risk screening and multifactorial prevention strategies (5). Another example using an electronic network for reaching a broad audience is found in Europe.

Falls Free Coalition

An example of an effective coalition is the Falls Free Coalition coordinated in the USA; a collective of representatives of national organizations and state coalitions working to reduce the growing number of falls and fall-related injuries among older adults (17). With support from the Archstone Foundation and Home Safety Council non-profit organizations, members of the Falls Free Coalition first convened in 2004 to write the Falls Free National Action Plan (4). The plan outlines key strategies and action plans for fall prevention to address the following five priority areas:

- physical mobility;

- medications management;

- home safety;

- environmental safety in the community; and

- cross-cutting issues, such as advocacy, policy, links to health care systems and integration of interdisciplinary activities.

More information about the National Action Plan, and the Coalition and its bimonthly newsletter may be found at www.healthyagingprograms.org.

c) Education

Along with good leadership and collaboration, education is an essential strategy for building the necessary capacity for effective fall prevention policy and practice. Such education is needed by those who:

- are at risk of falling;

- provide health and social services to those at risk; and

- are responsible for the design and construction of housing and public spaces used by older persons.

To be effective, education must be part of a larger strategy for falls prevention that reflects current evidence, adult learning principles and integration of learning to practice. An example of an education programme that reflects these principles is the Canadian Falls Prevention Curriculum.

ProFaNE

The Prevention of Falls Network Europe (ProFaNE) is a European community-funded thematic network to promote effective practice in falls prevention among older persons (6). With over 1100 website members from over 30 countries, an active discussion board, and nearly 900 resources, ProFaNE disseminates good practice by making all its resources publicly available at www.PROFANE.eu.org.

The Canadian Falls Prevention Curriculum ©

The Canadian Falls Prevention Curriculum© (7), funded by the Population Health Fund of the Public Health Agency of Canada is designed to provide community leaders and those who provide health and social services to older persons with the necessary skills to design, implement and evaluate evidence-based falls prevention programmes. To ensure relevance to the target audience the process for the development, testing and dissemination of the curriculum actively involves partners representing older persons, policy-makers, educators, researchers and health and social service providers. See www.injuryresearch.bc.ca for further information.

2. Prevention

There has been a substantial increase in the past decade in research on the prevention of falls among older persons. Considerable evidence now exists that most falls among older persons are associated with identifiable and modifiable risk factors and that targeted prevention efforts are shown to be cost-effective (9, 10, 11, 12). Most falls and resulting injuries among older persons are shown to result from a combination of age and disease-related conditions and the individual's interaction with their social and physical environment (9). It is also known that risk is greatly increased for those with multiple risk factors (11). There is good evidence to show that some interventions are more effective than others and those when tailored to individual risk profiles in community, residential and acute care settings are most effective.

Fallproof ©

Fallproof© is a comprehensive balance and mobility training programme designed for physical activity instructors and health professionals to build the necessary skills to reduce the risk of falling among community-based older adults (8). Based on a sound understanding of the physiology of ageing, adult learning theory and falls-prevention evidence, this programme provides instruction for the practical application of mobility and balance assessment and intervention.

a) Community

For older persons living in the community, evidence shows that health and environment risk-factor assessment with interventions based on assessment results, is highly effective in reducing falls among community-dwelling older persons who are cognitively intact (13, 14). Components of successful multifactorial approaches include:

- balance and gait training with appropriate use of assistive devices;

- environmental risk assessment and modification;

- medication review and modification;

- managing visual problems;

- providing education and training;

- addressing foot and shoe problems; and

- addressing orthostatic hypotension and other cardiovascular problems (12, 13, 14).

Exercise is shown to be an important component of a multifactorial intervention, particularly when applied consistently for ten weeks or longer (12). However, little is known about the cost effectiveness of exercise programmes for older persons and more research is necessary to determine the optimal type, duration, frequency and intensity of those programmes (15).

Within a multifactorial approach, the components of successful health interventions focus on post-fall clinical assessment followed by treatment involving a multidisciplinary-team approach. The following medical conditions are most often reported as target areas for fall reduction:

- cardiac dysrhythmias and orthostatic hypotension;

- reducing the number of medications, particularly those that contribute to postural hypotension or sedation;

- addressing gait and balance problems with appropriate assistive devices;

- rehabilitation for weakness and mobility problems;

- vitamin D and calcium supplementation; and

- treatment of correctable vision, particularly early cataract surgery (9, 10).

Environmental screening and modification programmes are shown to be most effective when they involve a multidisciplinary team and are targeted to those with a history of falling or known-risk factors (14). The precise components of successful home modification are not clearly understood. Most programmes target the removal hazards such as loose rugs, clutter electrical cords, unstable furniture and installation of bathroom grab bars, raised toilet seats, handrails on both sides of stairways and the use of personal alarm systems to call for help when necessary (9).

Evidence also exists to show that education and self-management programmes when used on their own without measures to implement change are not effective in the community setting (12).

While less effective that multifactorial approaches, there are a number of single-factor interventions shown to have a strong effect in reducing falls among community-dwelling older persons. Single interventions that are most strongly recommended include: exercise, home hazard assessment and modification, withdrawal of psychotropic medications, and cardiac pacing for fallers with carotid sinus hypersensitivity (13, 14).

As a single intervention strategy, the exercise approach shown to be most effective is individually tailored muscle strength and balance retraining prescribed by a trained-health professional.

Group exercise programmes are shown to be less effective than individually pre-scribed exercises with the exception of a group programme using the Tai Chi intervention – a form of Chinese martial arts (16).

b) Residential settings[1]:

As with community settings, multifactorial approaches are shown to be the most effect-prevention strategy in residential settings.

Components of successful multifactorial interventions include: staff training and guidance, changes in medication, resident education, environmental assessment and modification, supply and repair of aids, exercise, and use of hip protectors (12, 17, 10).

A single intervention shown to be effective in residential settings is the use of vitamin D and calcium supplements. Other single strategies that show promise include:

- gait training and advice on appropriate use of assistive devices;

- review and modification of medications, particularly psychotropics;

- nutritional review and supplementation;

- staff education programmes;

- exercise programmes;

- environmental modification;

- post-fall problem-solving sessions; and

- the use of hip protectors (12, 17).

There is no evidence to support the effectiveness of interventions to reduce falls among residents with cognitive impairments (17).

---

1   Residential setting: refers to nursing homes, care homes or long-term facilities

c) Acute care settings[2]:

No evidence exists to support the effectiveness of multifactorial interventions in acute care settings (14). The use of physical or pharmaceutical restraints commonly used with the intention of reducing falls is shown not to be effective. Conversely, there is moderate evidence to support an increased risk of injury from a fall with the use of restraints (12). Alternatives to restrains (lower bed, mats on floor, training on exercise and safe transfers) have moderate evidence for their effectiveness (12). Other interventions that have been tested but lack strong supporting evidence include: hospital discharge risk assessment and planning, exercise programmes, environmental modifications, use of bed alarms and the use of identification bracelets (18, 19). Some evidence exists to support facilitated home assessments for those at high risk for falling when discharged from hospital (10).

---

2   Acute care setting: refers to hospitals or rehabilitation units

3. Practice – Interventions

Practice settings are where falls prevention evidence is translated into feasible, affordable and sustainable interventions. Practitioners are well placed to link the application of evidence to organizational policies and to identify gaps that need to be addressed before successful adoption is possible. An effective tool for enacting the translation of evidence into practice is the development of a clinical practice guideline. An example of an effective guideline is produced by the Registered Nursing Association of Ontario (RNAO), Canada.

In less developed countries the translation of falls prevention evidence to practice is made difficult by competing demands for urgent health-care issues and shortages of health-care providers. In addition, before effective adoption of evidence to practice, more studies are necessary to better understand the unique contributors to falls among older people in less developed countries, including the influence of diet, hazardous environments, the lack of accessible safety equipment and transportation, and the role of inadequate health services.

The RNAO Prevention of Falls and Fall Injuries in the Older Adult Best Practice Guideline

The RNAO Prevention of Falls and Fall Injuries in the Older Adult Best Practice Guideline was designed for long-term and acute-care nurses to enhance their skills and abilities for risk assessment and prevention. The purpose of this guideline is to increase all nurses' confidence, knowledge, skills and abilities in the identification of adults within health-care facilities at risk of falling and to define interventions for the prevention of falling (20).

Injury outcomes among older persons in less developed versus more developed countries also need to be explored, particularly given that hip fractures are being described as an "orthopedic epidemic" in less developed countries [Baker et al;1992: cited in (21)].

4. Concluding remarks

Given recent rapid population ageing worldwide, without concerted action by policy-makers, researchers and practitioners, the economic and societal burden of falls will increase by epidemic proportions in all parts of the world over the next few decades. The complex and multifactorial nature of falls in older age demands a proactive and systematic approach to prevention. Healthy public policies and proven prevention strategies that are tailored to target populations are essential for the successful integration of fall-prevention evidence into practice for effective fall-risk identification and reduction.

5. References

1. Scott VJ, Peck S, Kendall P (2004). Prevention of falls and injuries among the elderly: a special report from the office of the provincial health officer. Victoria, British Colombia, Provincial Health Office, B.C. Ministry of Health.

2. British Columbia Injury Research and Prevention Unit (BCIRPU) (2006). Vancouver, British Columbia, (http://www.injuryresearch. bc.ca/, accessed 27 August 2007).

3. Herman M, Gallagher E, Scott VJ (2006). The evolution of seniors' falls prevention in British Columbia. Victoria, British Columbia, B.C. Ministry of Health, (http://www.health.gov. bc.ca/library/publications/year/2006/falls_ report.pdf, accessed 27 August 2007).

4. National Council on Aging (NCOA) Center for healthy aging model health programs for communities (2007). Washington, DC, Center for Health Aging (http:// healthyagingprograms.org/content. asp?sectionid=69, accessed 27 August 2007).

5. Fall Prevention Center of Excellence. Falls Free (2007). Washington, DC, Center for Healthy Aging (http://www.stopfalls.org/, accessed 27 August 2007).

6. Prevention of Falls Network Europe, ProFaNE (2007). Manchester, GB, ProFaNE (http://www.profane.eu.org/, accessed 27 August 2007).

7. Scott VJ et al. Canadian Falls Prevention Curriculum©, Vancouver, British Columbia. B.C. Injury Research and Prevention Unit, (unpublished data).

8. Rose, DJ (2003). Fallproof! A comprehensive balance and mobility training program. Windsor, Ontario, Human Kinetics.

9. Rubenstein LZ (2006). Falls in older people: epidemiology, risk factors and strategies for prevention. Age Ageing, 35-S2:ii37-ii41.

10. Rubenstein LZ et al. (2006). The summary of the newly updated ABS/BGS guideline: Evidence based practice guideline for the prevention of falls in older persons. Chicago: American Geriatrics Society Plenary Symposium, May 4, 2006.

11. Tinetti ME, Speechley M, Ginter SF (1988). Risk factors for falls among elderly persons living in the community. *New England Journal of Medicine*, 319(26):1701-1707.

12. Skelton D, Todd C (2004). What are the main risk factors for falls amongst older people and what are the most effective interventions to prevent these falls? Copenhagen, WHO Regional Office for Europe, Health Evidence Network report (http://www.euro.who.int/document/E82552.pdf, accessed 27 August 2007).

13. Chang JT et al. (2004). Interventions for the prevention of falls in older adults: systematic review and meta-analysis of randomised clinical trials. *British Medical Journal*, 328:680-683.

14. Gillespie LD et al. (2004). Interventions for preventing falls in elderly people. Cochrane Database of Systematic Reviews, (4):CD000340.

15. Gardner MM, Robertson MC, Campbell AJ. (2000). Exercise in preventing falls and fall related injuries in older people: a review of randomised controlled trials. *British Journal of Sports Medicine*, 1(34):7-17.

16. Wolf SL et al. (2003). Selected as the best paper in the 1990s: Reducing frailty and falls in older persons: An investigation of tai chi and computerized balance training. *Journal of the American Geriatrics Society*, 51(12):1794-1803.

17. Kannus P et al. (2000). Prevention of hip fracture in elderly people with use of a hip protector. *New England Journal of Medicine*, 343(21):1506-1513.

18. Hill K et al. (2000). An analysis of research on preventing falls and falls injury in older people: community, residential care and hospital settings (2004 update). Canberra, Australia, National Ageing Research Institute for the Commonwealth Department of Health and Aged Care.

19. Oliver D, Hopper A, Seed P (2000). Do hospital fall prevention programs work? A systematic review. *Journal of the American Geriatrics Society*, 48(12):1679-1689.

20. Registered Nurses' Association of Ontario (2005). Prevention of falls and fall injuries in the older adult. Toronto, Ontario, Registered Nurses' Association of Ontario (www.rnao.org/bestpractices/PDF/BPG_Falls_rev05.pdf, accessed 27 August 2007).

21. Barss P et al. (1998). Injury prevention: An international perspective. Epidemiology, surveillance, and policy. New York, Oxford, Oxford University Press.

22. World Health Organization (2002). Active ageing: A policy framework. Geneva.

Chapter VI. WHO Falls Prevention Model within the Active Ageing Framework

This chapter provides a summary of the preceding section of this document and presents the WHO Falls Prevention model within the Active Ageing Framework (see Figure 6 below). This model describes a cohesive, multisectoral approach to falls prevention that is built on the WHO Active Ageing Policy Framework – a proactive and flexible public health policy grounded in the principles of health promotion and disease prevention. Thus, the model recognizes the importance of a commitment to active ageing strategies and programmes that are designed to enhance the health, participation, and security of older people (see Chapter 2). The WHO vision of active ageing proposes strategies, interventions, and programmes that recognize the rights, needs, preferences and contributions of older people – and these are reflected in this model.

1. The need

Although population ageing is one of humanity's greatest triumphs, it also presents today's societies with one of their most significant challenges. Worldwide, the proportion of people age 60 and over is growing faster than any other age group. By 2050, the number of persons over the age of

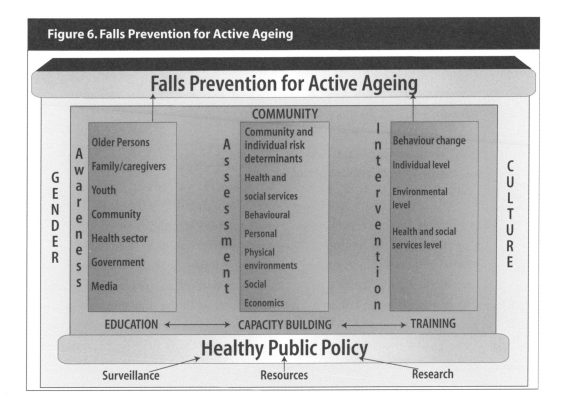

Figure 6. Falls Prevention for Active Ageing

60 years is expect to increase to more than two billion with 85% of them living in developing countries. Global ageing will place increased economic and social demands worldwide. However, the ageing population should not be viewed as a threat or a crisis. On the contrary, the WHO Active Ageing Framework recognizes that older persons are precious and invaluable resources who make an extraordinarily important contribution to the fabric of all societies.

A major factor behind the global ageing and the increase in life expectancy observed in most countries has been the impressive development of public health practices and policies that have greatly reduced premature deaths through the partial control of many previously fatal-infectious diseases. The worldwide development and implementation of PHC practices and the control of communicable diseases are important components of the WHO mission. This unfinished agenda has now been followed by a shift in the global burden of disease from the management of acute conditions to addressing the steady increase in noncommunicable diseases (NCDs). As individuals and societies age, NCDs are increasingly becoming the leading causes of morbidity, disability and mortality in all regions of the world.

Fortunately, many NCDs can be prevented through the application of appropriate health promotion and disease-prevention strategies. The WHO Active Ageing Framework recognizes that the failure to prevent or manage the growth of NCDs appropriately will result in enormous human and social costs. This would result in the inappropriate use of resources, which are still needed to address other health and social challenges. There is a need to shift the public health paradigm from one that focuses on "finding and fixing" acute problems to a more systematic, coordinated, and comprehensive strategy designed to prevent, treat, and manage the growing number of NCDs worldwide. The WHO Falls Prevention Model is an example of such a systematic, coordinated, and comprehensive strategy designed to reduce the burden of one of the most significant causes of age-related injuries and non-communicable conditions associated with old age.

The extensive reviews of the scientific literature summarized in earlier sections of this report underscore the reality that falls among older people are a large and increasing cause of injury, treatment costs and death in virtually all regions of the world. The WHO Active Ageing Framework recognizes that the injuries sustained as a consequence of a fall in old age are almost always more severe than when that occurs earlier in life.

For injuries of the same severity, older people experience more disability, longer hospital stays, extended periods of rehabilitation, a higher risk of subsequent dependency as well as a higher risk of dying. The good news is that many fall-related injuries are preventable. There is now compelling evidence that risk-factors for falling can be influenced by the implementation of targeted intervention strategies designed to modify the various intrinsic and extrinsic determinants known to increase the likelihood of falling. The WHO Falls Prevention Model provides a comprehensive multisectoral framework for reducing falls and fall-related injuries among older persons. The model is designed to identify policies, practices and procedures that will:

- build **awareness** of the importance of falls prevention and treatment among older persons;

- improve the **assessment** of individual, environmental, and societal factors that increase the likelihood of falls;

- facilitate the design and implementation of culturally-appropriated evidence-based **interventions** that will significantly reduce the number of falls among older persons.

2. The foundation

The WHO Falls Prevention Model within the Active Ageing Framework cannot succeed unless it is integrated into a healthy-public policy that embraces a multisectoral approach to the prevention, treatment, and management of NCDs. The WHO vision of healthy and active ageing requires the mobilization and commitment of many sectors of society including health and social services, education, employment and labour, finance, social security, housing, transportation, and both rural and urban development. Furthermore, all effective active-ageing policies and programmes realize the involvement of older people and their caregivers in all aspects of the planning, implementation and evaluation.

An effective falls-prevention strategy will need to acknowledge the cultural reality of the society in which it is to be implemented. The culture that surrounds all individuals and communities shapes and influences all of the determinants of active ageing. Cultural values and traditions determine not only how a given society views older people and the ageing process, but also the types of prevention, detection and treatment services that are most likely to be successful in a particular country and culture.

In order to address the diversity of cultural determinants, the WHO Falls Prevention Model requires the cross-national, transregional and global sharing of information and ideas. The Active Ageing Framework reminds us that all effective NCD prevention and treatment strategies will need to be firmly grounded within the local, national, and regional reality. These realities must consider factors such as epidemiological transition, rapid changes in the health sector, globalization, urbanization, changing family patterns and environmental degradation, as well as persistent inequalities and poverty, particularly in developing countries where the majority of older persons are already living.

The WHO Active Ageing Framework recognizes that effective policies and programmes designed to combat NCDs in old age need to adopt a life course perspective that acknowledges that most determinants of chronic conditions and disabilities have their roots in childhood as well as in young and middle-aged adult life. If a substantive decrease in the impact of falls on the health and quality of life of older persons is to be achieved, it will be necessary to develop programmes and policies that create supportive environments, reduce risk factors and foster healthy choices at all stages of the life course.

Any effective falls prevention strategy will also need to acknowledge the reality that globally, women are at greater risk for falls and fall-related injuries than men. Accordingly, gender issues need to be considered in the development of all policies, programmes and practices. The WHO Active Ageing Framework reminds us that in many societies, girls and women have lower social status and less access to food, education, meaningful work and health services. Because the consequences of falls disproportionately impact older women it is especially important that these factors be addressed proactively and explicitly within the Falls Prevention for Active Ageing context. Moreover, it is also important to observe that mortality rates resulting from injuries caused by falls are higher among older men than women of same age for reasons that are not yet fully understood. More research in this regard is urgently needed.

Finally, falls prevention policies and programmes cannot be targeted at only one level of determinants or risk-factors. Effective strategies will need to acknowledge and balance multiple levels of determinants including recognizing the importance of individual-level risk factors and responsibilities; the development of age-friendly and enabling environments; and the formulation of policies and programmes that maximize participation and inclusion of older persons.

The WHO Falls Prevention Model is built around three pillars that are highly interrelated and mutually dependent;

(1) Building awareness of the importance of falls prevention and treatment;

(2) Improving the assessment of individual, environmental and societal factors that increase the likelihood of falls; and

(3) Facilitating the design and implementation of culturally-appropriated evidence-based interventions that will significantly reduce the number of falls among older persons.

Making progress in implementing the strategies identified in each of these pillars will require an ongoing commitment to capacity building, education, and training in all countries and regions.

3. Three pillars of the WHO Falls Prevention Model:

a) Pillar One - Building awareness of the importance of falls prevention:

There is a need to build awareness of the importance of falls within all sectors of society that are impacted by falls and fall-related injuries. Awareness building is not restricted to educating individuals and groups about the significance of falls as modifiable risk factors for disabling conditions and increased mortality. It also involves education about the increasing economic and social costs associated with the failure to address falls and fall-risk factors in a systematic manner. **Awareness** will need to be built within the following constituencies:

Older persons: Any strategy to build awareness of the importance of falls and fall prevention must begin with older persons themselves. Many of them are unaware that falls are preventable. In many cultures falling is considered to be a normal, unavoidable consequence of growing older. The WHO Active Ageing Framework calls for increasing basic-health education and health literacy through a commitment to lifelong learning about health and disease prevention. By applying such an approach to educating older adults about falls and fall prevention, not only would older adults become more aware of the importance of paying close attention to fall-related risk factors and determinants but they would also be more likely to take action to correct these challenges to their health and independence.

Family and caregivers: Both informal and formal caregivers have a critical role to play in building awareness about the importance of falls and falls prevention. It is especially important to provide family members, peer counsellors and other informal caregivers with information and training on how to identify risk factors for falls and how to take action to decrease the likelihood of falling among those at greatest risk. It is also critical to ensure that formal caregivers are fully familiar with the latest evidence related to the assessment, prevention, and treatment of falls. This will comprise the incorporation of modules on falls and fall prevention in professional caregiver curricula at all levels, including continuing education. Within the developing world, it is important to acknowledge the contribution of healers who are knowledgeable about alternative and complementary medicines. These individuals should be encouraged to integrate their special skills and knowledge with contemporary evidence-based practice related to falls and fall prevention.

Youth and young adults: Any active-ageing strategy that strives to be effective in reducing the prevalence of chronic diseases and disabling conditions will need to adopt a life course perspective. This is especially important in the area of falls and falls prevention because many of the individual-level determinants, which predispose a person to be at risk for injurious falls, begin to manifest themselves early in life. Furthermore, building awareness of the importance of falls and fall-related issues in children and youth will increase the likelihood to implementing intergenerational approaches to falls prevention and treatment.

Community: The majority of older persons grow old in their own homes and in the communities they have lived in for most of their lives. Accordingly, it is important to educate all sectors of these communities about the importance of a proactive, evidence-based strategy for reducing falls. Building awareness of risk factors for falls at the community level is particularly important because there is evidence that the structure of the physical environment can impact the likelihood of an older person to fall. It can also make the difference between independence and dependence for individuals who live in unsafe environments or areas with multiple physical barriers. These barriers can render older persons more susceptible to isolation, depression, reduced physical activity, and increased mobility problems.

Health sector:: The WHO Active Ageing Framework recognizes that building awareness and changing the attitudes of health and social-service providers is paramount to ensuring that their practices enable and empower individuals to remain as autonomous and independent as doable for as long as possible. Within the area of falls and falls prevention, health professionals have a critical role to play in identifying risk factors and determinants for falls, and for recommending culturally-appropriated evidence base interventions for the prevention, treatment and management of falls

and fall-related injuries. It is important to provide incentives and training for health and social service professionals. This will increase their awareness and understanding of contemporary research and practices so that they are able to counsel healthy lifestyle practices that reduce falls and fall-related injuries among men and women of all ages.

Government: Raising awareness of the importance of falls prevention among government officials at all levels is critical if the resources and other support needed to implement a comprehensive, multisectoral fall prevention strategy at any of societal levels are to be made available. It is important to underscore that a commitment to prevention and treatment of falls is both cost-effective and the right thing to do. Legislators and government officials should be invited to participate in all aspects of the development and implementation of public health policies and practices that focus on health promotion and disease prevention.

Media: The media have an important role to play in promoting a positive image of ageing, therefore building awareness among them of the significance of falls and falls prevention is paramount. The media can help by widely disseminating realistic and positive images of active ageing, as well as by sharing educational information on falls and falls prevention strategies. The media can also help to confront negative stereotypes about growing old and help to combat persistent ageism.

b) Pillar Two – Improving the identification and assessment of risk factors and determinants of falls:

There is a growing appreciation that a complex combination of individual-level, community-wide, and societal factors influence the probability of falls and fall-related injuries among older persons. Although the evidence base regarding how best to identify and assess the various risk factors and determinants for falls is growing, there are many areas where information is lacking and improvements are needed. A systematic multisectoral strategy for reducing falls and fall-related injuries will require concerted efforts to improve **assessment** and identify critical determinants in each of the following domains:

Health and social services: Convenient and affordable access to health and social services can greatly impact an older persons' likelihood of experiencing a fall or fall-related injury. Health and social services should be structured in such a way as to routinely screen older persons for known-risk factors for falls. Health professionals should be trained to use evidence-based protocols and procedures that help to identify those individuals who are at the greatest risk. Suitable follow-up strategies should be in place to assist clinicians to recommend culturally-appropriated and affordable evidence-based treatment programmes when indicated. The WHO Active Ageing Framework notes that health and social services need to be integrated, coordinated and cost-effective.

Furthermore, there must be neither age nor gender discrimination in the provision of services and service providers should treat people of all ages with dignity and respect.

Behavioural: : There is a growing appreciation that a number of important behavioural factors impact older persons vulnerability to falls and their likelihood to seek treatment or care for falls and fall-related conditions. Many older adults incorrectly believe that it is too late to change their behaviour and adopt a healthy lifestyle in old age. Others experience a significant fear of falling that greatly limits their activity choices, reduces their independence and decreases their engagement in society. It is not sufficient to simply educate older adults about the importance of falls and falls prevention, it is also crucial to assess their readiness to change their lifestyles and adopt preventative and/or rehabilitative therapies. Any integrated strategy to reduce falls at the individual and/or community level will need to acknowledge and assess the critical behavioural determinants known to impact an individual's risk for falling. Attention to these factors can significantly increase the chance that a person will engage in appropriate preventive behaviours such as physical activity, healthy eating, not smoking and using alcohol and medications wisely. These behaviours can in turn help to prevent disease and functional decline, extend longevity and enhance quality of life.

Personal: There are many personal or individual-level risk factors and determinants that can influence an individual's likelihood of experiencing a fall. In any comprehensive falls prevention programme, effective evidence-based strategies will need to be developed to screen for and identify individual-level risk factors known to be associated with an increased risk for falling. The specific nature of such screening protocols will inevitably vary as a function of the resources and expertise available to perform these assessments. At the most basic level, evidence-based questionnaires are available to screen older persons for key risks factors. Ideally, more comprehensive clinical examinations can be used to assess for known risk factors such as physical inactivity, decreased muscle strength, impaired balance, poor vision, confusion, inadequate or inappropriate medication and/or polypharmacy. Accurate identification of individual-level risk factors and determinants can greatly increase the likelihood of selecting an appropriate prevention or treatment strategy that is targeted to meet the needs of the individual older person.

Physical environments: There is a growing appreciation that the nature and structure of the physical environment can significantly influence the likelihood of an individual to suffer a fall or fall-related injury. The WHO Active Ageing Framework underscores the need to ensure that the older-people physical environments are "age-friendly" because this can make a difference between independence and dependence. There is a growing base of knowledge suggesting that a systematic assessment of and attention to environmental risk factors such as unsafe sidewalks, poorly lit roadways, and inaccessible or unsafe neighborhoods can significantly increase the likelihood of falls among older persons. There are also many risk factors within the homes, in which older people live, that place them at an increased risk for falling. In many countries home-safety visits have proved to be effective for identifying environmental risks factors that increase the risk of falling. The need to address environmental determinants of falls may be particularly acute in developing countries where many older persons are forced to live in arrangements that are not of their choice, such as with relatives in already crowded households. In many developing countries, the proportion of older people living in slums and shanty towns is rising rapidly. Older people living in these settlements are at an increased risk for falls and fall-related injuries.

Social: Older persons who have suffered from fall-related injuries and others who experience a fear of falling can often become isolated and disengaged from the community. Any comprehensive falls prevention programme will need to recognize and acknowledge the critical role that social support plays in providing opportunities for older persons to fully participate in society. The WHO Active Ageing Framework recognizes that opportunities for education and lifelong learning, peace, and protection from violence and abuse are key factors in the social environment that enhance health, participation and security as people age. Loneliness, social isolation, illiteracy and a lack of education, abuse and exposure to conflict situations greatly increase older people's risks for disabilities and early death. Inadequate social support is associated not only with an increase in mortality, morbidity and psychological distress but a decrease in overall health and well-being. Assessment of and attention to the adequacy of social support in an older person's environment is an important element of a comprehensive fall-risk assessment protocol and can make a difference between success and failure of an intervention strategy.

Economic: The economic environment, in which an older person lives, can play a profound impact on their health and quality of life. The WHO Active Ageing Framework reminds us that economic factors such as income, work and social protection need to be considered when developing effective strategies in the area of active ageing. All ageing policies must acknowledge the reality of poverty and the impact that a lot of lack of personal resources has on the opportunities available to an older person. Active-ageing policies need to intersect with broader schemes to reduce poverty at all ages. While all poor people face an increased risk of ill-health and disabilities, older people are particularly vulnerable. In many countries and cultures, older people are, by necessity or choice, continuing to work in the labour force well into old age. Others participate in unpaid labour through childcare and work within the home and in the fields. Continued employment of older persons can be a "double-edged sword".

On the one hand, it provides opportunities for older persons to earn money and stay active and engaged in the community, on the other it can place older persons at increased risk for accident and injury, particularly in cases where the worksite is hazardous with inadequate facilities and lighting.

In all countries, families provide the majority of support for older people who require help. However, as societies develop and the tradition of generations living together declines, mechanisms that provide social protection for older people who are unable to earn a living and are alone and vulnerable are needed. National, regional, and local falls-prevention strategies cannot be developed independently of these cultural, political, and economic realities?.

c) Pillar Three - Identifying and implementing realistic and effective interventions

Falls are complex events that are caused by a combination of intrinsic impairments and disabilities which are often compounded by a variety of environmental hazards. Due to the multifactorial nature of falls risk factors and determinants, numerous studies have shown that **interventions** can be effective in reducing falls in older people by simultaneously targeting several intrinsic and extrinsic risk factors or determinants. Successful multifaceted-intervention programmes have included such components as:

- medical assessment;

- home safety checks and advice;

- monitoring of prescription medications;

- environmental changes;

- tailored exercise and physical activity;

- training in transfer skills and gait;

- assessment of readiness to change behaviour; and

- referral of clients to health-care professionals.

Unfortunately, multifactorial falls prevention interventions can be labour-intensive and expensive both for the individual and the community. For these reasons, decisions regarding whether to implement a comprehensive, multifaceted falls-prevention intervention, or targeted interventions addressing individual risk factors and determinants will need to be made at the local or national level. These shown-effective decisions need to take into account a variety of economic, cultural, and political factors. In the section below, information about some of the most promising interventions that have been shown to be effective in reducing the incidence of falls and fall-related injuries in older populations is summarized.

Behaviour change: In recent years growing attention has focused on the study of behavioural factors that increase the probability of an individual in initiating and maintaining an intervention designed to promote health and/or reduce the risk of chronic conditions. There is now good evidence that incorporating a comprehensive behavioural change strategy into interventions designed to increase health and well-being can help to maximize recruitment, increase motivation, and minimize attrition. Among the behavioural strategies that have been shown to increase the likelihood that a person will sustain a new behaviour are the following:

- Securing social support from family and friends.

- Promoting the participant's self-efficacy and perceived competence.

- Providing older persons with active choices that are tailored to their personal needs and preferences.

- Encouraging older persons to commit to an intervention by developing health contracts and/or goal statements that include realistic and measurable plans of action with specified health goals.

- Concerns for safety are identified as a barrier to changing behaviour by many older adults. Educating participants about actual risks of interventions can help to alleviate many of these concerns.

- Providing regular and accurate performance feedback can assist older adults in developing realistic expectations about their own progress.

- Positive reinforcement strategies increase the likelihood of maintenance of an activity. Examples of effective-reinforcement strategies include recruitment incentives, rewards for reaching targeted goal, and public recognition for attendance and adherence.

Environmental modification: There is now good evidence that home-hazard assessment and modification that is professionally prescribed for older persons with a history of falling is effective in reducing risk. However, the value of home visits and home-hazard assessments in low-risk populations is less clear. Among the factors addressed in a typical-home visit include the assessment and improvement of lighting, the identification and removal of rugs and other trip hazards, and the installation of railings on staircases in bathrooms and toilets. The value of systematic hazard assessment and intervention has also been shown to be effective in decreasing falls in retirement homes and seniors centers where large numbers of individuals with elevated risk live or regularly visit.

There is growing interest in examining the impact of community level interventions designed to identify and correct environmental hazards that reduce physical and social activity and increase the risk of older persons falling. Among the environmental hazards assessed in environmental audits and "walkability" assessments are: unsafe sidewalks, poorly lit roadways, and inaccessible or unsafe neighborhoods. Although evidence of the impact of environmental changes on the incidence of falls and the number of fall-related injuries is insufficient to draw definitive conclusions, these interventions show promise and additional research is necessary to shed more light on the relationship between environmental changes and both fall risk and actual falls.

Health management: There is good evidence that access to appropriate and affordable medical care can significantly impact health and quality of life as well as decrease the likelihood of developing noncommunicable diseases. Because older people are more likely to suffer from a variety of chronic conditions, their access to medical care is especially important and can make the difference between early detection and timely intervention, and delayed and/or non-existent treatment and care. In the area of falls prevention, the accurate identification of individuals at high risk for falling is an important element in the selection of the evidence-based intervention with the greatest chance of a positive outcome. There is evidence that identifying patients who attend accident and emergency departments after falls, and referring them for subsequent therapy significantly reduces subsequent falls.

Older persons are more likely than younger people to need and use medications. Unfortunately, medications are often either unavailable or over-prescribed in this population. Averse drug-related reactions, polypharmacy, and confusion induced by psychotropic medication are all associated with an increased risk of falls and fall-related injuries. Health care strategies that require regular and systematic review of prescription and over-the counter medications have been shown to decrease the number of falls in older adult populations. Because visual impairments, especially poor contrast sensitivity and poor depth perception, have been shown to be significant risk factors for falling and fall-induced injuries, regular visual examinations with appropriate follow-up as necessary can be beneficial in reducing falls in older adults.

Physical activity: The WHO Heidelberg Guidelines for Physical Activity for Older Persons recommend that virtually all older persons should participate in physical activity on a regular basis. There are well established physiological, psychological, and social benefits associated with participation in physical activity. Furthermore, regular physical activity is associated with a significant decrease in risk for most non-communicable diseases. With respect to falls prevention, regular physical activity has been shown to prevent and/or lower an older person's risk for falling in community and home settings.

For healthy older adults at low risk for falls, engaging in a broad range of physical activities on a regular basis is likely to be sufficient to substantially reduce the risk of falling.

In contrast, older adults at higher risk for falls will benefit from engaging in structured exercise programmes that systematically target the risk factors amenable to change and are progressed at a rate that is determined by the individual's capabilities and previous experience with physical activity. Older adults identified at the highest risk for falls will benefit from an individually-tailored exercise programme that is embedded within a larger multifactorial intervention approach. In these populations, regular strength and balance exercises, such as, Tai Chi programmes have been shown to be effective in reducing the risk of both non-injurious and injurious falls. Additional research is necessary to quantify the optimum type, frequency, duration, and intensity of exercise needed to produce the maximum benefit. Because regular physical activity provides substantial health-related benefits and it is cheap, safe, and readily available, it is likely that physical activity programmes will play a major role in the prevention, treatment, and management of falls in most countries and cultures.

4. The way forward:

The WHO Falls Prevention for Active Ageing model provides an action plan for making progress in reducing the prevalence of falls in the older adult population. By building on the three pillars of falls prevention, the model proposes specific strategies for:

1. building awareness of the importance of falls prevention and treatment;

2. improving the assessment of individual, environmental, and societal factors that increase the likelihood of falls; and

3. for facilitating the design and implementation of culturally-appropriate, evidence-based interventions that will significantly reduce the number of falls among older persons.

The model provides strategies and solutions that will require the engagement of multiple sectors of society. It is dependent on and consistent with the vision articulated in the WHO Active Ageing Policy Framework. Although not all of the awareness, assessment, and intervention strategies identified in the model apply equally well in all regions of the world, there are significant evidence-based strategies that can be effectively implemented in all regions and cultures. The degree to which progress will be made depends on to the success in integrating falls prevention strategies into the overall health and social care agendas globally. In order to do this effectively, it is necessary to identify and implement culturally appropriate, evidence-based policies and procedures. This requires multisectoral collaborations, strong commitment to public and professional education, interaction based on evidence drawn from a variety of traditional, complementary, and alternative sources. Although the understanding of the evidence-base is growing, there is much that is not yet understood. Thus, there is an urgent need for continued research in all areas of falls prevention and treatment in order to better understand the scope of the problem worldwide. In particular, more evidence of the cost-effectiveness of interconnections is needed to develop strategies that are most likely to be effective in specific setting and population sub-groups.

While this is an ambitious plan, it is attainable. A tangible difference in the health and quality of life of older people around the world could be achieved by implementing a comprehensive global strategy to reduce falls.